Mediterran

Diet C   ҡ

20

50 Healthy and Tasty
Recipes to Kickstart your
Health Goals

By Stella Romero

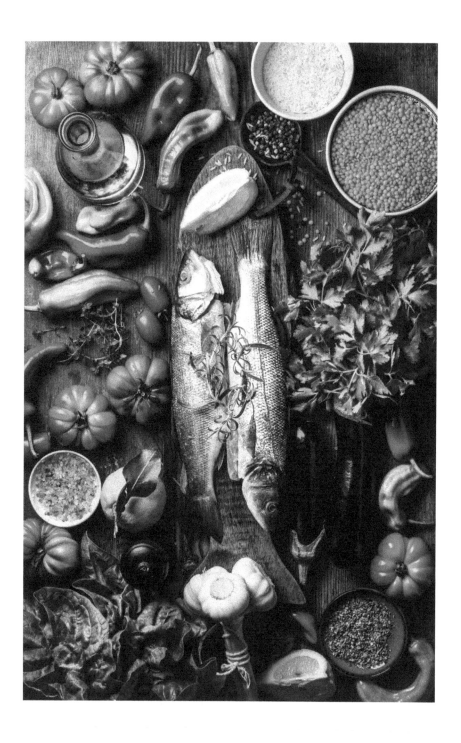

Table of Contents

Chapter 7: Dessert Recipes 100

with the express written consent from the Publisher. All additional right reserved.

The information in the following pages is broadly considered a truthful and accurate account of facts and as such, any inattention, use, or misuse of the information in question by the reader will render any resulting actions solely under their purview. There are no scenarios in which the publisher or the original author of this work can be in any fashion deemed liable for any hardship or damages that may befall them after undertaking information described herein.

Additionally, the information in the following pages is intended only for informational purposes and should thus be thought of as universal. As befitting its nature, it is presented without assurance regarding its prolonged validity or interim quality. Trademarks that are mentioned are done without written consent and can in no way be considered an endorsement from the trademark holder.

Introduction

Mediterranean diet is based on the eating habits of the inhabitants of the regions along the Mediterranean Sea, mostly from Italy, Spain and Greece; it is considered more a life style then a diet, in fact it also promotes physical activity and proper liquid (mostly water) consumption.

Depending on fresh seasonal local foods there are no strict rules, because of the many cultural differences, but there are some common factors.

Mediterranean diet has become famous for its ability to reduce heart disease and obesity, thanks to the low consumption of unhealthy fats that increase blood glucose.

Mediterranean diet is mostly plant based, so it's rich of antioxidants; vegetables, fruits like apple and grapes, olive oil, whole grains, herbs, beans and nuts are consumed in large quantities.

Moderate amounts of poultry, eggs, dairy and seafood are also common aliments, accompanied by a little bit of red wine (some studies say that in small amount it helps to stay healthy).
Red meat and sweets like cookies and cakes are accepted but are more limited in quantity.

Foods to avoid:

- refined grains, such as white bread and pasta
- dough containing white flour refined oils (even canola oil and soybean oil)
- foods with added sugars (like pastries, sodas, and candies)
- processed meats processed or packaged foods

Chapter 1: Breakfast and Snack Recipes

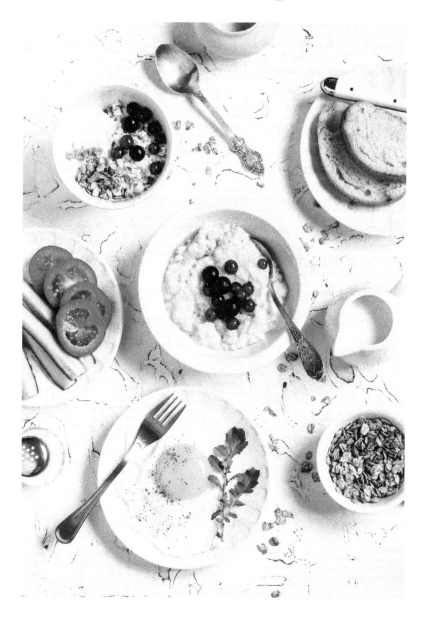

Shrimp Toast

Servings: 4 | Cooking: 10 min

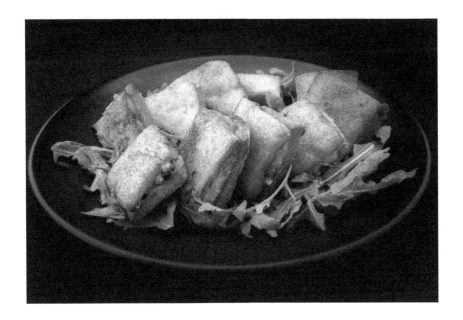

Ingredients

- 13 oz shrimps, peeled
- 1 tablespoon tomato sauce
- ½ teaspoon Splenda
- ¼ teaspoon garlic powder
- 1 teaspoon fresh parsley, chopped
- ½ teaspoon olive oil
- 1 teaspoon lemon juice
- 4 whole-grain bread slices

- 1 cup water, for cooking

Directions

1. Pour water in the saucepan and bring it to boil.
2. Add shrimps and boil them over the high heat for 5 minutes.
3. After this, drain shrimps and chill them to the room temperature.
4. Mix up together shrimps with Splenda, garlic powder, tomato sauce, and fresh parsley.
5. Add lemon juice and stir gently.
6. Preheat the oven to 360F.
7. Brush the bread slices with olive oil and bake for 3 minutes.
8. Then place the shrimp mixture on the bread. Bruschetta is cooked.

Nutrition: calories 199; fat 3.7; fiber 2.1; carbs 15.3; protein 24.1

Breakfast Beans (ful Mudammas)

Servings: 1 Cup | Cooking: 10 min

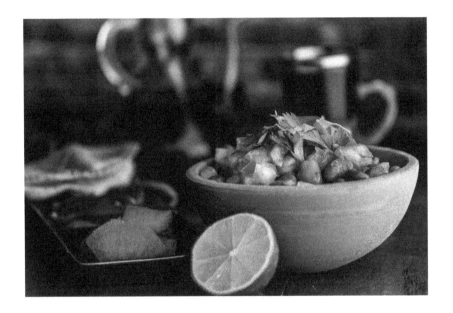

Ingredients

- 1 (15-oz.) can chickpeas, rinsed and drained
- 1 (15-oz.) can fava beans, rinsed and drained
- 1 cup water
- 1 TB. minced garlic
- 1 tsp. salt
- 1/2 cup fresh lemon juice
- 1/2 tsp. cayenne
- 1/2 cup fresh parsley, chopped

- 1 large tomato, diced
- 3 medium radishes, sliced
- 1/4 cup extra-virgin olive oil

Directions

1. In a 2-quart pot over medium-low heat, combine chickpeas, fava beans, and water. Simmer for 10 minutes.
2. Pour bean mixture into a large bowl, and add garlic, salt, and lemon juice. Stir and smash half of beans with the back of a wooden spoon.
3. Sprinkle cayenne over beans, and evenly distribute parsley, tomatoes, and radishes over top. Drizzle with extra-virgin olive oil, and serve warm or at room temperature.

Seeds And Lentils Oats

Servings: 4 | Cooking: 50 min

Ingredients

- ½ cup red lentils
- ¼ cup pumpkin seeds, toasted
- 2 teaspoons olive oil
- ¼ cup rolled oats
- ¼ cup coconut flesh, shredded
- 1 tablespoon honey
- 1 tablespoon orange zest, grated
- 1 cup Greek yogurt
- 1 cup blackberries

Directions

1. Spread the lentils on a baking sheet lined with parchment paper, introduce in the oven and roast at 370 degrees F for 30 minutes.
2. Add the rest of the ingredients except the yogurt and the berries, toss and bake at 370 degrees F for 20 minutes more.

3. Transfer this to a bowl, add the rest of the ingredients, toss, divide into smaller bowls and serve for breakfast.

Nutrition: calories 204; fat 7.1; fiber 10.4; carbs 27.6; protein 9.5

Couscous With Artichokes, Sun-dried Tomatoes And Feta

Servings: 6 | Cooking: 15 min

Ingredients

- 3 cups chicken breast, cooked, chopped
- 2 1/3 cups water, divided
- 2 jars (6-ounces each) marinated artichoke hearts, undrained
- 1/4 teaspoon black pepper, freshly ground
- 1/2 cup tomatoes, sun-dried
- 1/2 cup (2 ounces) feta cheese, crumbled
- 1 cup flat-leaf parsley, fresh, chopped
- 1 3/4 cups whole-wheat Israeli couscous, uncooked
- 1 can (14 1/2 ounces) vegetable broth

Directions

1. In a microwavable bowl, combine 2 cups of the water and the tomatoes. Microwave on HIGH for about 3 minutes or until the water boils. When water is boiling, remove from the microwave,

cover, and let stand for about 3 minutes or until the tomatoes are soft; drain, chop, and set aside.

2. In a large saucepan, place the vegetable broth and the remaining 1/3 cup of water; bring to boil. Stir in the couscous, cover, reduce heat, and simmer for about 8 minutes or until tender.

3. Remove the pan from the heat; add the tomatoes and the remaining ingredients. Stir to combine.

Nutrition:419 Cal, 14.1 g total fat (3.9 g sat. fat, 0.8 g poly. Fat, 1.4 g mono), 64 mg chol.,677 mg sodium, 42.5 g carb.,2.6 g fiber, 30.2 g protein.

Cinnamon Roll Oats

Servings: 4 | Cooking: 10 min

Ingredients

- ½ cup rolled oats
- 1 cup milk
- 1 teaspoon vanilla extract
- 1 teaspoon ground cinnamon
- 2 teaspoon honey
- 2 tablespoons Plain yogurt
- 1 teaspoon butter

Directions

1. Pour milk in the saucepan and bring it to boil.
2. Add rolled oats and stir well.
3. Close the lid and simmer the oats for 5 minutes over the medium heat. The cooked oats will absorb all milk.
4. Then add butter and stir the oats well.
5. In the separated bowl, whisk together Plain yogurt with honey, cinnamon, and vanilla extract.
6. Transfer the cooked oats in the serving bowls.

7. Top the oats with the yogurt mixture in the shape of the wheel.

Nutrition: Calories 243; fat 20.2; fiber 1; carbs 2.8; protein 13.3

Mediterranean Wrap

Servings: 4 | Cooking: 10 min

Ingredients

- 4 pieces (10-inch) spinach wraps (or whole wheat tortilla or sun-dried tomato wraps)
- 1 pound chicken tenders
- 1 cup cucumber, chopped
- 3 tablespoons extra-virgin olive oil
- 1 medium tomato, chopped
- 1/3 cup couscous, whole-wheat
- 2 teaspoons garlic, minced
- 1/4 teaspoon salt, divided
- 1/4 teaspoon freshly ground pepper
- 1/4 cup lemon juice
- 1/2 cup water
- 1/2 cup fresh mint, chopped
- 1 cup fresh parsley, chopped

Directions

1. In a small saucepan, pour the water and bring to a boil. Stir in the couscous, remove pan from heat,

cover, and allow to stand for 5 minutes, then fluff using a fork; set aside.

2. Meanwhile, in a small mixing bowl, combine the mint, parsley, oil, lemon juice, garlic, 1/8 teaspoon of the salt, and the pepper.

3. In a medium mixing bowl, toss the chicken with the 1 tablespoon of the mint mixture and the remaining 1/8 teaspoon of salt.

4. Place the chicken mixture into a large non-stick skillet; cook for about 3-5 minutes each side, or until heated through. Remove from the skillet, allow to cool enough to handle, and cut into bite-sized pieces.

5. Stir the remaining mint mixture, the cucumber, and the tomato into the couscous.

6. Spread about 3/4 cup of the couscous mix onto each wrap and divide the chicken between the wraps, roll like a burrito, tucking the sides in to hold to secure the ingredients in. Cut in halves and serve.

Nutrition:479 Cal, 17 g total fat (3 g sat. fat, 11 g mono), 67 mg chol., 653 mg sodium, 382 pot., 49 g carb.,5 g fiber, 15 g protein.

Chicken Liver

Servings: ¾ Cup | Cooking: 7 min

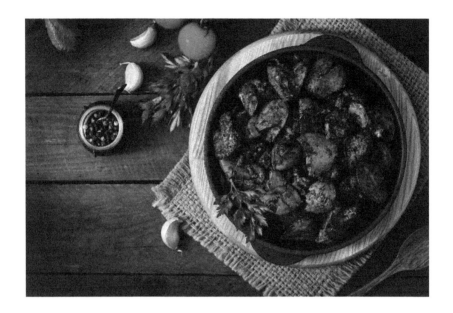

Ingredients

- 2 lb. chicken liver
- 3 TB. extra-virgin olive oil
- 3 TB. minced garlic
- 1 tsp. salt
- 1/2 tsp. ground black pepper
- 1 cup fresh cilantro, finely chopped
- 1/4 cup fresh lemon juice

Directions

1. Cut chicken livers in half, rinse well, and pat dry with paper towels.
2. Preheat a large skillet over medium heat. Add extra-virgin olive oil and garlic, and cook for 2 minutes.
3. Add chicken liver and salt, and cook, tossing gently, for 5 minutes. Remove the skillet from heat, and spoon liver onto a plate.
4. Add black pepper, cilantro, and lemon juice. Lightly toss, and serve warm.

Avocado Spread

Servings: 8 | Cooking: 0 min

Ingredients

- 2 avocados, peeled, pitted and roughly chopped
- 1 tablespoon sun-dried tomatoes, chopped
- 2 tablespoons lemon juice
- 3 tablespoons cherry tomatoes, chopped
- ¼ cup red onion, chopped
- 1 teaspoon oregano, dried
- 2 tablespoons parsley, chopped
- 4 kalamata olives, pitted and chopped
- A pinch of salt and black pepper

Directions

1. Put the avocados in a bowl and mash with a fork.
2. Add the rest of the ingredients, stir to combine and serve as a morning spread.

Nutrition: calories 110; fat 10; fiber 3.8; carbs 5.7; protein 1.2

Eggs with Zucchini Noodles

Preparation: 10 min | Cooking: 11 min | Servings: 2

Ingredients

- 2 tablespoons extra-virgin olive oil
- 3 zucchinis, cut with a spiralizer
- 4 eggs
- A pinch of red pepper flakes
- 1 tablespoon basil, chopped

Directions

1. In a bowl, combine the zucchini noodles with salt, pepper and the olive oil and toss well.
2. Grease a baking sheet using cooking spray and divide the zucchini noodles into 4 nests on it.
3. Whisk an egg on top of each nest, sprinkle salt, pepper and the pepper flakes on top then bake at 350 F for 11 min.
4. Divide the mix between plates, sprinkle the basil on top and serve.

Nutrition: 296 calories; 23g fat; 3.3g fiber;

Banana Oats

Preparation: 10 min | Cooking: 0 min | Servings: 2

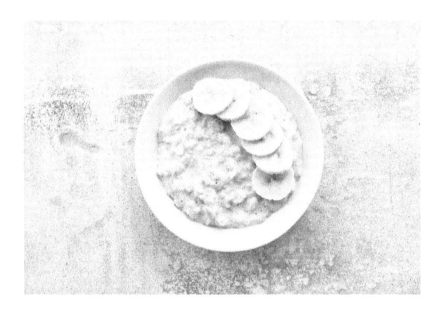

Ingredients

- ½ cup cold brewed coffee
- 2 dates, pitted
- 2 tablespoons cocoa powder
- 1 cup rolled oats
- 1 and ½ tablespoons chia seeds

Directions

1. In a blender, combine the 1 banana with the ¾ almond milk and the rest of the ingredients, pulse, divide into bowls and serve for breakfast.

Nutrition: 451 calories; 25g fat; 9.9g fiber;

Chapter 2: Lunch & Dinner Recipes

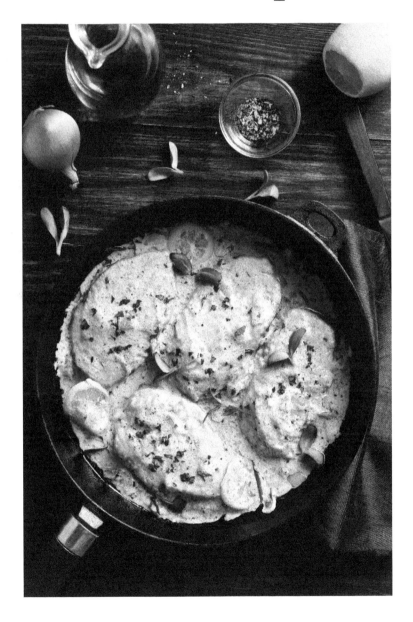

Spicy Tomato Poached Eggs

Servings: 4 | Cooking: 30 min

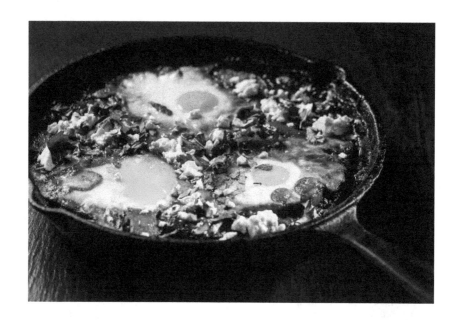

Ingredients

- 2 tablespoons olive oil
- 2 shallots, chopped
- 2 garlic cloves, chopped
- 2 red bell peppers, cored and sliced
- 2 yellow bell peppers, cored and sliced
- 2 tomatoes, peeled and diced
- 1 cup vegetable stock
- 1 jalapeno, chopped

- Salt and pepper to taste
- 4 eggs

Directions

1. Heat the oil in a saucepan and stir in the shallots, garlic, bell peppers and jalapeno. Cook for 5 minutes.
2. Add the tomatoes, stock, thyme and bay leaf, as well as salt and pepper to taste.
3. Cook for 10 minutes on low heat.
4. Crack open the eggs and drop them in the hot sauce.
5. Cook on low heat for 5 additional minutes.
6. Serve the eggs and the sauce fresh and warm.

Nutrition: Calories:179 Fat:11.9g Protein:7.6g Carbohydrates:11.7g

Mediterranean Scones

Servings: 8 | Cooking: 15-20 min

Ingredients

- 1 egg, beaten, to glaze
- 1 tablespoon baking powder
- 1 tablespoon olive oil
- 1/4 tsp salt
- 10 black olives, pitted, halved
- 100 g feta cheese, cubed
- 300 ml full-fat milk
- 350 g self-rising whole-wheat flour
- 50 g butter, cut in pieces
- 8 halves Italian sundried tomatoes, coarsely chopped

Directions

1. Preheat the oven to 220C, gas to 7, or fan to 200C.
2. Grease a large-sized baking sheet with butter.
3. In a large mixing bowl, mix the flour, the baking powder, and the salt. Rub in the oil and the butter,

until the flour mix resembles fine crumbs. Add the cheese, tomatoes, and the olives.

4. Create a well in the center of the flour mix, pour the milk, and with a knife, mix using cutting movements, until the flour mixture is a stickyish, soft dough. Make sure that you do not over mix the dough.

5. Flour the work surface and your hands well; shape the dough into 3 to 4-cm think round. Cut into 8 wedges; place the wedges well apart in the prepared baking sheet. Brush the wedges with the beaten egg; bake for about 15-20 minutes, until the dough has risen, golden, and springy.

6. Transfer into a wire rack; cover with a clean tea towel to keep them soft.

7. Serve warm and buttered.

8. Store in airtight container for up to 2 to 3 days.

Nutrition:293 Cal, 14 g total fat (7 g sat. fat), 36 g carb.,0 g sugar, 2 g fiber, 8 g protein, and 2 g sodium.

Mixed Olives Braised Chicken

Servings: 4 | Cooking: 1 Hour

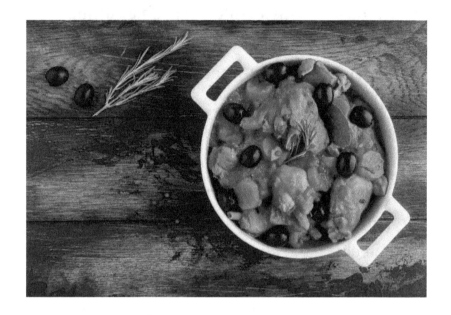

Ingredients

- 4 chicken breasts
- 2 shallots, sliced
- 4 garlic cloves, chopped
- 2 red bell peppers, cored and sliced
- ½ cup black olives
- ½ cup green olives
- ½ cup kalamata olives
- 2 tablespoons olive oil

- ¼ cup white wine
- ½ cup vegetable stock
- Salt and pepper to taste
- 1 bay leaf
- 1 thyme sprig

Directions

1. Combine the shallots, garlic, bell peppers, olives, oil, wine and stock in a deep dish baking pan.
2. Season with salt and pepper and place the chicken in the pan over the olives.
3. Cook in the preheated oven at 350F for 45 minutes.
4. Serve the chicken warm and fresh.

Nutrition: Calories:280 Fat:16.3g Protein:22.9g Carbohydrates:7.9g

Coconut Chicken Meatballs

Servings: 4 | Cooking: 10 min

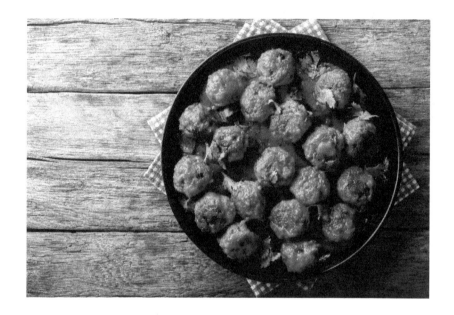

Ingredients

- 2 cups ground chicken
- 1 teaspoon minced garlic
- 1 teaspoon dried dill
- 1/3 carrot, grated
- 1 egg, beaten
- 1 tablespoon olive oil
- ¼ cup coconut flakes
- ½ teaspoon salt

Directions

1. In the mixing bowl mix up together ground chicken, minced garlic, dried dill, carrot, egg, and salt.
2. Stir the chicken mixture with the help of the fingertips until homogenous.
3. Then make medium balls from the mixture.
4. Coat every chicken ball in coconut flakes.
5. Heat up olive oil in the skillet.
6. Add chicken balls and cook them for 3 minutes from each side. The cooked chicken balls will have a golden brown color.

Nutrition: calories 200; fat 11.5; fiber 0.6; carbs 1.7; protein 21.9

Grilled Turkey With White Bean Mash

Servings: 4 | Cooking: 45 min

Ingredients

- 4 turkey breast fillets
- 1 teaspoon chili powder
- 1 teaspoon dried parsley
- Salt and pepper to taste
- 2 cans white beans, drained
- 4 garlic cloves, minced
- 2 tablespoons lemon juice
- 3 tablespoons olive oil
- 2 sweet onions, sliced
- 2 tablespoons tomato paste

Directions

1. Season the turkey with salt, pepper and dried parsley.
2. Heat a grill pan over medium flame and place the turkey on the grill. Cook on each side for 7 minutes.

3. For the mash, combine the beans, garlic, lemon juice, salt and pepper in a blender and pulse until well mixed and smooth.
4. Heat the oil in a skillet and add the onions. Cook for 10 minutes until caramelized. Add the tomato paste and cook for 2 more minutes.
5. Serve the grilled turkey with bean mash and caramelized onions.

Nutrition: Calories:337 Fat:8.2g Protein:21.1g Carbohydrates:47.2g

Chapter 3: Meat Recipes

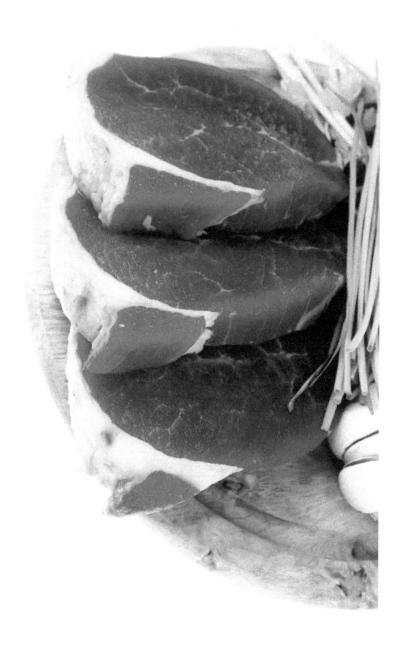

Rosemary Pork Chops

Servings: 4 | Cooking: 35 min

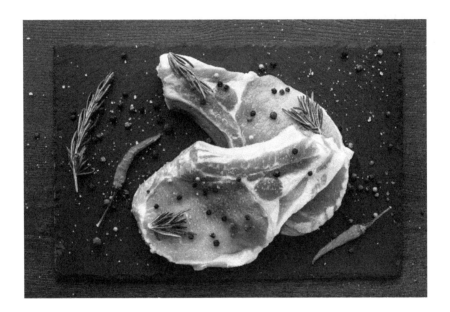

Ingredients

- 4 pork loin chops, boneless
- Salt and black pepper to the taste
- 4 garlic cloves, minced
- 1 tablespoon rosemary, chopped
- 1 tablespoon olive oil

Directions

1. In a roasting pan, combine the pork chops with the rest of the ingredients, toss, and bake at 425 degrees F for 10 minutes.
2. Reduce the heat to 350 degrees F and cook the chops for 25 minutes more.
3. Divide the chops between plates and serve with a side salad.

Nutrition: calories 161; fat 5; fiber 1; carbs 1; protein 25

Cauliflower Tomato Beef

Servings: 2 | Cooking: 25 min

Ingredients

- 1/2 lb beef stew meat, chopped
- 1 tsp paprika
- 1 tbsp balsamic vinegar
- 1 celery stalk, chopped
- 1/4 cup grape tomatoes, chopped
- 1 onion, chopped
- 1 tbsp olive oil
- 1/4 cup cauliflower, chopped
- Pepper
- Salt

Directions

1. Add oil into the instant pot and set the pot on sauté mode.
2. Add meat and sauté for 5 minutes.
3. Add remaining ingredients and stir well.
4. Seal pot with lid and cook on high for 20 minutes.
5. Once done, allow to release pressure naturally. Remove lid.

6. Stir and serve.

Nutrition: Calories 306 Fat 14.3 g Carbohydrates 7.6 g Sugar 3.5 g Protein 35.7 g Cholesterol 101 mg

Pork And Sour Cream Mix

Servings: 4 | Cooking: 40 min

Ingredients

- 1 and ½ pounds pork meat, boneless and cubed
- 1 red onion, chopped
- 1 tablespoon avocado oil
- 1 garlic clove, minced
- ½ cup chicken stock
- 2 tablespoons hot paprika
- Salt and black pepper to the taste
- 1 and ½ cups sour cream
- 1 tablespoon cilantro, chopped

Directions

1. Heat up a pot with the oil over medium heat, add the pork and brown for 5 minutes.
2. Add the onion and the garlic and cook for 5 minutes more.
3. Add the rest of the ingredients except the cilantro, bring to a simmer and cook over medium heat for 30 minutes.

4. Add the cilantro, toss, divide between plates and serve.

Nutrition: calories 300; fat 9.5; fiber 4.5; carbs 15.5; protein 22

Honey Pork Strips

Servings: 4 | Cooking: 8 min

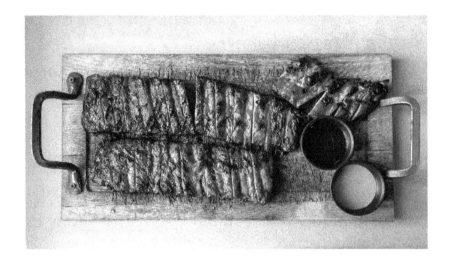

Ingredients

- 10 oz pork chops
- 1 teaspoon liquid honey
- 1 teaspoon tomato sauce
- 1 teaspoon sunflower oil
- ½ teaspoon sage
- ½ teaspoon mustard

Directions

1. Cut the pork chops on the strips and place in the bowl.
2. Add liquid honey, tomato sauce, sunflower oil, sage, and mustard.
3. Mix up the meat well and leave for 15-20 minutes to marinate.
4. Meanwhile, preheat the grill to 385F.
5. Arrange the pork strips in the grill and roast them for 4 minutes from each side. Sprinkle the meat with remaining honey liquid during to cooking to make the taste of meat juicier.

Nutrition: calories 245; fat 18.9; fiber 0.1; carbs 1.7; protein 16.1

Orange Lamb And Potatoes

Servings: 4 | Cooking: 7 Hours

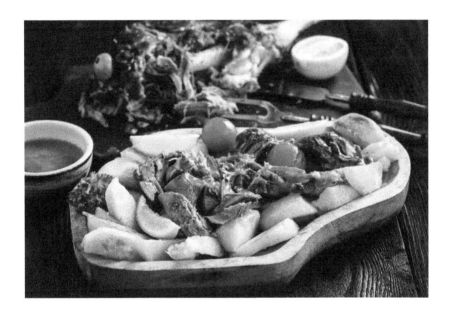

Ingredients

- 1 pound small potatoes, peeled and cubed
- 2 cups stewed tomatoes, drained
- Zest and juice of 1 orange
- 4 garlic cloves, minced
- 3 and ½ pounds leg of lamb, boneless and cubed
- Salt and black pepper to the taste
- ½ cup basil, chopped

Directions

1. In your slow cooker, combine the lamb with the potatoes and the rest of the ingredients, toss, put the lid on and cook on Low for 7 hours.
2. Divide the mix between plates and serve hot.

Nutrition: calories 287; fat 9.5; fiber 7.3; carbs 14.8; protein 18.2

Chapter 4: Poultry Recipes

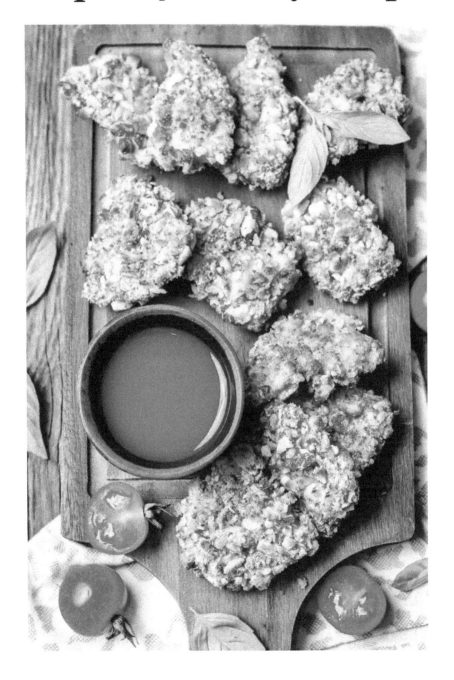

Parmesan Chicken

Servings: 3 | Cooking: 30 min

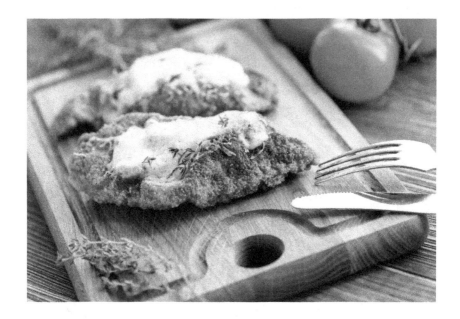

Ingredients

- 1-pound chicken breast, skinless, boneless
- 2 oz Parmesan, grated
- 1 teaspoon dried oregano
- ½ teaspoon dried cilantro
- 1 tablespoon Panko bread crumbs
- 1 egg, beaten
- 1 teaspoon turmeric

Directions

1. Cut the chicken breast on 3 servings.
2. Then combine together Parmesan, oregano, cilantro, bread crumbs, and turmeric.
3. Dip the chicken servings in the beaten egg carefully.
4. Then coat every chicken piece in the cheese-bread crumbs mixture.
5. Line the baking tray with the baking paper.
6. Arrange the chicken pieces in the tray.
7. Bake the chicken for 30 minutes at 365F.

Nutrition: calories 267; fat 9.5; fiber 0.5; carbs 3.2; protein 40.4

Pomegranate Chicken

Servings: 6 | Cooking: 25 min

Ingredients

- 1-pound chicken breast, skinless, boneless
- 1 tablespoon za'atar
- ½ teaspoon salt
- 1 tablespoon pomegranate juice
- 1 tablespoon olive oil

Directions

1. Rub the chicken breast with za'atar seasoning, salt, olive oil, and pomegranate juice.
2. Marinate the chicken or 15 minutes and transfer in the skillet.
3. Roast the chicken for 15 minutes over the medium heat.
4. Then flip the chicken on another side and cook for 10 minutes more.
5. Slice the chicken and place in the serving plates.

Nutrition: calories 107; fat 4.2; fiber 0; carbs 0.2; protein 16.1

Chicken With Artichokes And Beans

Servings: 4 | Cooking: 40 min

Ingredients

- 2 tablespoons olive oil
- 2 chicken breasts, skinless, boneless and halved
- Zest of 1 lemon, grated
- 3 garlic cloves, crushed
- Juice of 1 lemon
- Salt and black pepper to the taste
- 1 tablespoon thyme, chopped
- 6 ounces canned artichokes hearts, drained
- 1 cup canned fava beans, drained and rinsed
- 1 cup chicken stock
- A pinch of cayenne pepper
- Salt and black pepper to the taste

Directions

1. Heat up a pan with the oil over medium-high heat, add chicken and brown for 5 minutes.

2. Add lemon juice, lemon zest, salt, pepper and the rest of the ingredients, bring to a simmer and cook over medium heat for 35 minutes.
3. Divide the mix between plates and serve right away.

Nutrition: calories 291; fat 14.9; fiber 10.5; carbs 23.8; protein 24.2

Chicken Pie

Servings: 6 | Cooking: 50 min

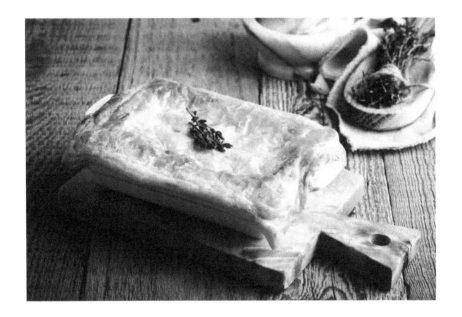

Ingredients

- ¼ cup green peas, frozen
- 1 carrot, chopped
- 1 cup ground chicken
- 5 oz puff pastry
- 1 tablespoon butter, melted
- ¼ cup cream
- 1 teaspoon ground black pepper
- 1 oz Parmesan, grated

Directions

1. Roll up the puff pastry and cut it on 2 parts.
2. Place one puff pastry part in the non-sticky springform pan and flatten.
3. Then mix up together green peas, chopped carrot, ground chicken, and ground black pepper.
4. Place the chicken mixture in the puff pastry.
5. Pour cream over mixture and sprinkle with Parmesan.
6. Cover the mixture with second puff pastry half and secure the edges of it with the help of the fork.
7. Brush the surface of the pie with melted butter and bake it for 50 minutes at 365F.

Nutrition: calories 223; fat 14.3; fiber 1; carbs 13.2; protein 10.5

Chicken And Semolina Meatballs

Servings: 8 | Cooking: 10 min

Ingredients

- 1/3 cup carrot, grated
- 1 onion, diced
- 2 cups ground chicken
- 1 tablespoon semolina
- 1 egg, beaten
- ½ teaspoon salt
- 1 teaspoon dried oregano
- 1 teaspoon dried cilantro
- 1 teaspoon chili flakes
- 1 tablespoon coconut oil

Directions

1. In the mixing bowl combine together grated carrot, diced onion, ground chicken, semolina, egg, salt, dried oregano, cilantro, and chili flakes.
2. With the help of scooper make the meatballs.
3. Heat up the coconut oil in the skillet.
4. When it starts to shimmer, put meatballs in it.

5. Cook the meatballs for 5 minutes from each side over the medium-low heat.

Nutrition: calories 102; fat 4.9; fiber 0.5; carbs 2.9; protein 11.2

Chapter 5: Fish and Seafood Recipes

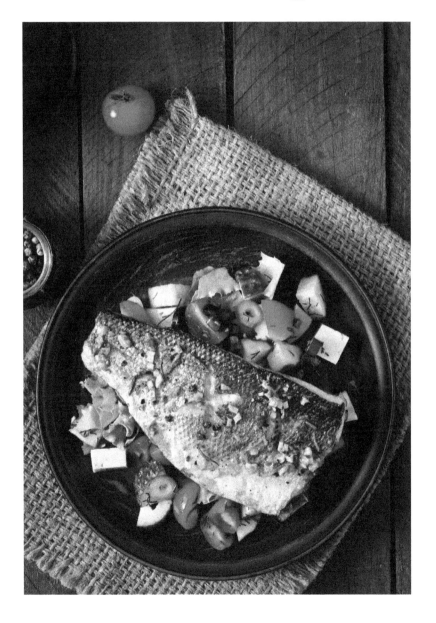

Kale, Beets And Cod Mix

Servings: 4 | Cooking: 20 min

Ingredients

- 2 tablespoons apple cider vinegar
- ½ cup chicken stock
- 1 red onion, sliced
- 4 golden beets, trimmed, peeled and cubed
- 2 tablespoons olive oil
- Salt and black pepper to the taste
- 4 cups kale, torn
- 2 tablespoons walnuts, chopped
- 1 pound cod fillets, boneless, skinless and cubed

Directions

1. Heat up a pan with the oil over medium-high heat, add the onion and the beets and cook for 3-4 minutes.
2. Add the rest of the ingredients except the fish and the walnuts, stir, bring to a simmer and cook for 5 minutes more.

3. Add the fish, cook for 10 minutes, divide between plates and serve.

Nutrition: calories 285; fat 7.6; fiber 6.5; carbs 16.7; protein 12.5

Shrimp Scampi

Servings: 6 | Cooking: 8 min

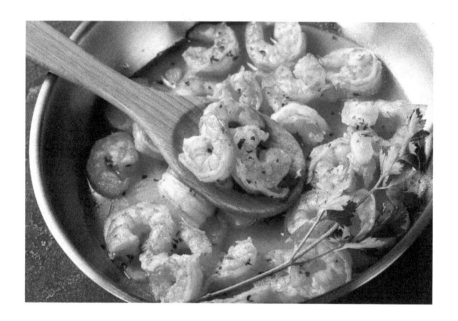

Ingredients

- 1 lb whole wheat penne pasta
- 1 lb frozen shrimp
- 2 tbsp garlic, minced
- 1/4 tsp cayenne
- 1/2 tbsp Italian seasoning
- 1/4 cup olive oil
- 3 1/2 cups fish stock
- Pepper

- Salt

Directions

1. Add all ingredients into the inner pot of instant pot and stir well.
2. Seal pot with lid and cook on high for 6 minutes.
3. Once done, release pressure using quick release. Remove lid.
4. Stir well and serve.

Nutrition: Calories 435 Fat 12.6 g Carbohydrates 54.9 g Sugar 0.1 g Protein 30.6 g Cholesterol 116 mg

Orange Rosemary Seared Salmon

Servings: 4 | Cooking: 10 min

Ingredients

- ½ cup chicken stock
- 1 cup fresh orange juice
- 1 tablespoon coconut oil
- 1 tablespoon tapioca starch
- 2 garlic cloves, minced
- 2 tablespoon fresh lemon juice
- 2 teaspoon fresh rosemary, minced
- 2 teaspoon orange zest
- 4 salmon fillets, skins removed
- Salt and pepper to taste

Directions

1. Season the salmon fillet on both sides.
2. In a skillet, heat coconut oil over medium high heat. Cook the salmon fillets for 5 minutes on each side. Set aside.
3. In a mixing bowl, combine the orange juice, chicken stock, lemon juice and orange zest.

4. In the skillet, sauté the garlic and rosemary for 2 minutes and pour the orange juice mixture. Bring to a boil. Lower the heat to medium low and simmer. Season with salt and pepper to taste.
5. Pour the sauce all over the salmon fillet then serve.

Nutrition: Calories: 493; Fat: 17.9g; Protein: 66.7g; Carbs: 12.8g

Salmon And Mango Mix

Servings: 2 | Cooking: 25 min

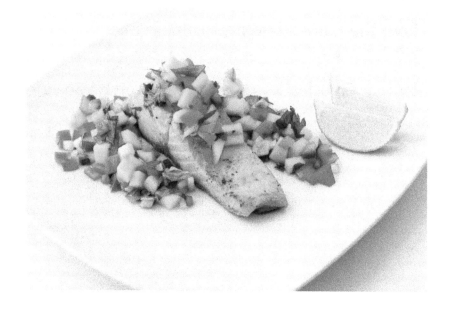

Ingredients

- 2 salmon fillets, skinless and boneless
- Salt and pepper to the taste
- 2 tablespoons olive oil
- 2 garlic cloves, minced
- 2 mangos, peeled and cubed
- 1 red chili, chopped
- 1 small piece ginger, grated
- Juice of 1 lime

- 1 tablespoon cilantro, chopped

Directions

1. In a roasting pan, combine the salmon with the oil, garlic and the rest of the ingredients except the cilantro, toss, introduce in the oven at 350 degrees F and bake for 25 minutes.
2. Divide everything between plates and serve with the cilantro sprinkled on top.

Nutrition: calories 251; fat 15.9; fiber 5.9; carbs 26.4; protein 12.4

Delicious Shrimp Alfredo

Servings: 4 | Cooking: 3 min

Ingredients

- 12 shrimp, remove shells
- 1 tbsp garlic, minced
- 1/4 cup parmesan cheese
- 2 cups whole wheat rotini noodles
- 1 cup fish broth
- 15 oz alfredo sauce
- 1 onion, chopped
- Salt

Directions

1. Add all ingredients except parmesan cheese into the instant pot and stir well.
2. Seal pot with lid and cook on high for 3 minutes.
3. Once done, release pressure using quick release. Remove lid.
4. Stir in cheese and serve.

Nutrition: Calories 669 Fat 23.1 g Carbohydrates 76 g Sugar 2.4 g Protein 37.8 g Cholesterol 190 mg

Chapter 6: Salads & Side Dishes

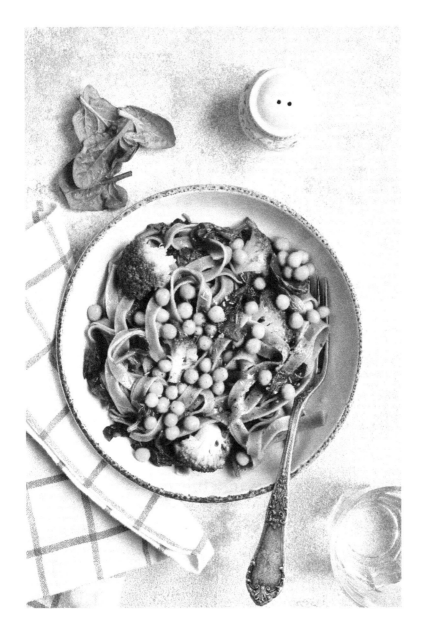

Grilled Veggie and Hummus Wrap

Preparation: 15 min | Cooking: 10 min | Servings: 6

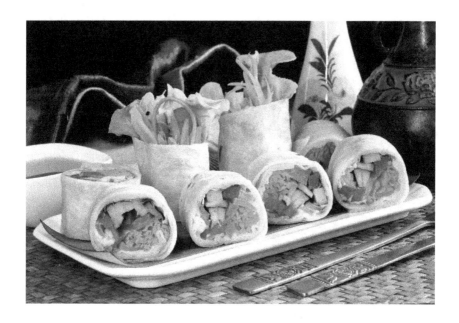

Ingredients

- 1 large eggplant
- 1 large onion
- ½ cup extra-virgin olive oil
- 6 lavash wraps or large pita bread
- 1 cup Creamy Traditional Hummus

Directions

1. Preheat a grill, large grill pan, or lightly oiled large skillet on medium heat.
2. Slice the eggplant and onion into circles. Rub the vegetables with olive oil and sprinkle with salt.
3. Cook the vegetables on both sides, about 3 to 4 min each side.
4. To make the wrap, lay the lavash or pita flat. Scoop 3 tablespoons of hummus on the wrap.
5. Evenly divide the vegetables among the wraps, layering them along one side of the wrap. Gently fold over the side of the wrap with the vegetables, tucking them in and making a tight wrap.
6. Lay the wrap seam side-down and cut in half or thirds.
7. You can also wrap each sandwich with plastic wrap to help it hold its shape and eat it later.

Nutrition: 362 Calories: 15g Protein: 28g Carbohydrates

Spanish Green Beans

Preparation: 10 min | Cooking: 20 min | Servings: 4

Ingredients

- 1 large onion, chopped
- 4 cloves garlic, finely chopped
- 1-pound green beans, fresh or frozen, trimmed
- 1 (15-ounce) can diced tomatoes

Directions

1. In a huge pot over medium heat, cook olive oil, onion, and garlic; cook for 1 minute.
2. Cut the green beans into 2-inch pieces.
3. Add the green beans and 1 teaspoon of salt to the pot and toss everything together; cook for 3 min.
4. Add the diced tomatoes, remaining ½ teaspoon of salt, and black pepper to the pot; continue to cook for another 12 min, stirring occasionally.
5. Serve warm.

Nutrition: 200 Calories: 4g Protein: 18g Carbohydrates

Roasted Cauliflower and Tomatoes

Preparation: 5 min | Cooking: 25 min | Servings: 4

Ingredients

- 4 cups cauliflower, cut into 1-inch pieces
- 6 tablespoons extra-virgin olive oil, divided
- 4 cups cherry tomatoes
- ½ teaspoon freshly ground black pepper
- ½ cup grated Parmesan cheese

Directions

1. Preheat the oven to 425°F.
2. Add the cauliflower, 3 tablespoons of olive oil, and ½ teaspoon of salt to a large bowl and toss to evenly coat. Fill onto a baking sheet and arrange the cauliflower out in an even layer.
3. In another large bowl, add the tomatoes, remaining 3 tablespoons of olive oil, and ½ teaspoon of salt, and toss to coat evenly. Pour onto a different baking sheet.
4. Put the sheet of cauliflower and the sheet of tomatoes in the oven to roast for 17 to 20 min until the cauliflower is lightly browned and tomatoes are plump.

5. Using a spatula, spoon the cauliflower into a serving dish, and top with tomatoes, black pepper, and Parmesan cheese. Serve warm.

Nutrition: 294 Calories: 9g Protein: 13g Carbohydrates

Rustic Cauliflower and Carrot Hash

Preparation: 10 min | Cooking: 10 min | Servings: 4

Ingredients

- 1 large onion, chopped
- 1 tablespoon garlic, minced
- 2 cups carrots, diced
- 4 cups cauliflower pieces, washed
- ½ teaspoon ground cumin

Directions

1. Using big skillet over medium heat, cook 3 tbsps. of olive oil, onion, garlic, and carrots for 3 min.
2. Cut the cauliflower into 1-inch or bite-size pieces. Add the cauliflower, salt, and cumin to the skillet and toss to combine with the carrots and onions.
3. Cover and cook for 3 min.
4. Throw the vegetables and continue to cook uncovered for an additional 3 to 4 min.
5. Serve warm.

Nutrition: 159 Calories: 3g Protein: 15g Carbohydrates

Roasted Acorn Squash

Preparation: 10 min | Cooking: 35 min | Servings: 6

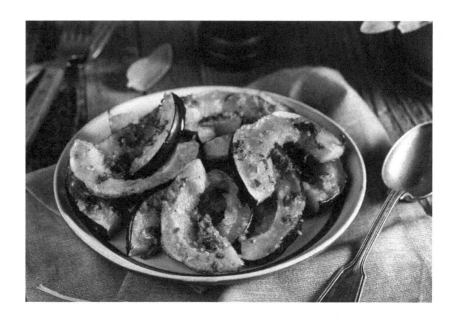

Ingredients

- 2 acorn squash, medium to large
- 2 tablespoons extra-virgin olive oil
- 5 tablespoons unsalted butter
- ¼ cup chopped sage leaves
- 2 tablespoons fresh thyme leaves

Directions

1. Preheat the oven to 400°F.

2. Cut the acorn squash in half lengthwise. Scoop out the seeds and cut it horizontally into ¾-inch-thick slices.
3. In a large bowl, drizzle the squash with the olive oil, sprinkle with salt, and toss together to coat.
4. Lay the acorn squash flat on a baking sheet.
5. Situate the baking sheet in the oven and bake the squash for 20 min. Flip squash over with a spatula and bake for another 15 min.
6. Cook the butter in a medium saucepan over medium heat.
7. Sprinkle the sage and thyme to the melted butter and let them cook for 30 seconds.
8. Transfer the cooked squash slices to a plate. Spoon the butter/herb mixture over the squash. Season with salt and black pepper. Serve warm.

Nutrition: 188 Calories: 1g Protein: 16g Carbohydrates

Sweet Veggie-Stuffed Peppers

Preparation: 20 min | Cooking: 30 min | Servings: 6

Ingredients

- 6 large bell peppers, different colors
- 3 cloves garlic, minced
- 1 carrot, chopped
- 1 (16-ounce) can garbanzo beans
- 3 cups cooked rice

Directions

1. Preheat the oven to 350°F.
2. Make sure to choose peppers that can stand upright. Cut off the pepper cap and remove the seeds, reserving the cap for later. Stand the peppers in a baking dish.
3. In a skillet over medium heat, cook up olive oil, 1 onion, garlic, and carrots for 3 min.
4. Stir in the garbanzo beans. Cook for another 3 min.
5. Take out the pan from the heat and spoon the cooked ingredients to a large bowl.
6. Add the rice, salt, and pepper; toss to combine.

7. Stuff each pepper to the top and then put the pepper caps back on.
8. Wrap the baking dish using aluminum foil and bake for 25 min.
9. Pull out the foil and bake for 6 min.
10. Serve warm.

Nutrition: 301 Calories: 8g Protein: 50g Carbohydrate

Sautéed Garlic Spinach

Preparation: 5 min | Cooking: 10 min | Servings: 4

Ingredients

¼ cup extra-virgin olive oil

1 large onion, thinly sliced

3 cloves garlic, minced

6 (1-pound) bags of baby spinach, washed

1 lemon, cut into wedges

Direction

Cook the olive oil, onion, and garlic in a large skillet for 2 min over medium heat.

Add one bag of spinach and ½ teaspoon of salt. Cover the skillet and let the spinach wilt for 30 seconds.

Repeat (omitting the salt), adding 1 bag of spinach at a time.

When all is added, open and cook for 3 min, letting some of the moisture evaporate.

Serve warm with lemon juice over the top.

Nutrition: 301 Calories: 17g Protein: 29g Carbohydrates

Garlicky Sautéed Zucchini with Mint

Preparation: 5 min | Cooking: 10 min | Servings: 4

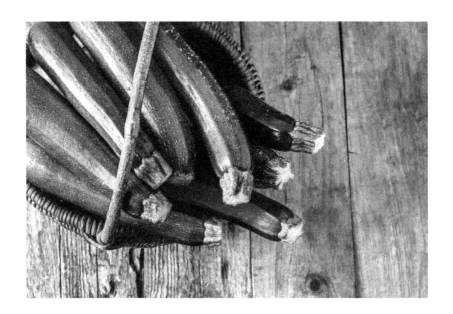

Ingredients

- 3 large green zucchinis
- 3 tablespoons extra-virgin olive oil
- 1 large onion, chopped
- 3 cloves garlic, minced
- 1 teaspoon dried mint

Directions

1. Cut the zucchini into ½-inch cubes.

2. Using huge skillet, place over medium heat, cook the olive oil, onions, and garlic for 3 min, stirring constantly.

3. Add the zucchini and salt to the skillet and toss to combine with the onions and garlic, cooking for 5 min.

4. Add the mint to the skillet, tossing to combine. Cook for another 2 min. Serve warm.

Nutrition: 147 Calories: 4g Protein: 12g Carbohydrates

Stewed Okra

Preparation: 5 min | Cooking: 25 min | Servings: 4

Ingredients

- 4 cloves garlic, finely chopped
- 1 pound fresh or frozen okra, cleaned
- 1 (15-ounce) can plain tomato sauce
- 2 cups water
- ½ cup fresh cilantro, finely chopped

Directions

1. In a big pot at medium heat, stir and cook ¼ cup of olive oil, 1 onion, garlic, and salt for 1 minute.
2. Stir in the okra and cook for 3 min.
3. Add the tomato sauce, water, cilantro, and black pepper; stir, cover, and let cook for 15 min, stirring occasionally.
4. Serve warm.

Nutrition: 201 Calories: 4g Protein: 18g Carbohydrates

Moussaka

Preparation: 55 min | Cooking: 40 min | Servings: 6

Ingredients

- 2 large eggplants, onions
- 10 cloves garlic, sliced
- 2 (15-ounce) cans diced tomatoes
- 1 (16-ounce) can garbanzo beans
- 1 teaspoon dried oregano

Directions

1. Slice the eggplant horizontally into ¼-inch-thick round disks. Sprinkle the eggplant slices with 1 teaspoon of salt and place in a colander for 31min.
2. Preheat the oven to 450°F. Pat the slices of eggplant dry with a paper towel and spray each side with an olive oil spray or lightly brush each side with olive oil.
3. Spread eggplant in a layer on a baking sheet. Bake for 10 min.
4. With a spatula, turn it over and bake for 12 min.
5. Using big skillet add the olive oil, onions, garlic, and remaining 1 teaspoon of salt. Cook for 3 min.

Add the tomatoes, garbanzo beans, oregano, and black pepper. Simmer for 11 min.

6. Using a deep casserole dish, begin to layer, starting with eggplant, then the sauce. Repeat until all ingredients have been used. Bake in the oven for 20 min.

7. Remove from the oven and serve warm.

Nutrition: 262 Calories: 8g Protein: 35g Carbohydrates

Bulgur Tomato Pilaf

Servings: 1 Cup | Cooking: 27 min

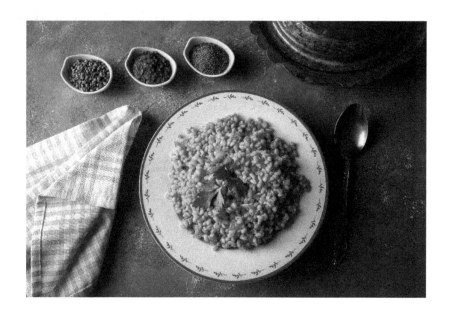

Ingredients

- 1 lb. ground beef
- 3 TB. extra-virgin olive oil
- 1 large yellow onion, finely chopped
- 2 medium tomatoes, diced
- 11/2 tsp. salt
- 1 tsp. ground black pepper
- 2 cups plain tomato sauce
- 2 cups water

- 2 cups bulgur wheat, grind

Directions

1. In a large, 3-quart pot over medium heat, brown beef for 5 minutes, breaking up chunks with a wooden spoon.
2. Add extra-virgin olive oil and yellow onion, and cook for 5 minutes.
3. Stir in tomatoes, salt, and black pepper, and cook for 5 minutes.
4. Add tomato sauce and water, and simmer for 10 minutes.
5. Add bulgur wheat, and cook for 2 minutes. Remove from heat, cover, and let sit for 5 minutes. Uncover, fluff bulgur with a fork, cover, and let sit for 5 more minutes.
6. Serve warm.

Garbanzo And Kidney Bean Salad

Servings: 4 | Cooking: 0 min

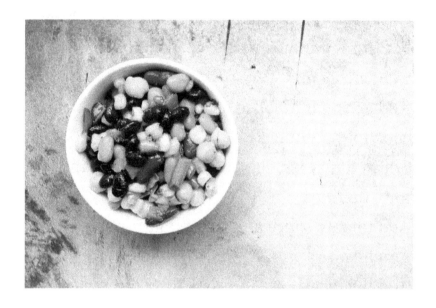

Ingredients

- 1 (15 ounce) can kidney beans, drained
- 1 (15.5 ounce) can garbanzo beans, drained
- 1 lemon, zested and juiced
- 1 medium tomato, chopped
- 1 teaspoon capers, rinsed and drained
- 1/2 cup chopped fresh parsley
- 1/2 teaspoon salt, or to taste
- 1/4 cup chopped red onion

- 3 tablespoons extra virgin olive oil

Directions

1. In a salad bowl, whisk well lemon juice, olive oil and salt until dissolved.
2. Stir in garbanzo, kidney beans, tomato, red onion, parsley, and capers. Toss well to coat.
3. Allow flavors to mix for 30 minutes by setting in the fridge.
4. Mix again before serving.

Nutrition: Calories per serving: 329; Protein: 12.1g; Carbs: 46.6g; Fat: 12.0g

Rice & Currant Salad Mediterranean Style

Servings: 4 | Cooking: 50 min

Ingredients

- 1 cup basmati rice
- salt
- 2 1/2 Tablespoons lemon juice
- 1 teaspoon grated orange zest
- 2 Tablespoons fresh orange juice
- 1/4 cup olive oil
- 1/2 teaspoon cinnamon
- Salt and pepper to taste
- 4 chopped green onions
- 1/2 cup dried currants
- 3/4 cup shelled pistachios or almonds
- 1/4 cup chopped fresh parsley

Directions

1. Place a nonstick pot on medium high fire and add rice. Toast rice until opaque and starts to smell, around 10 minutes.

2. Add 4 quarts of boiling water to pot and 2 tsp salt. Boil until tender, around 8 minutes uncovered.
3. Drain the rice and spread out on a lined cookie sheet to cool completely.
4. In a large salad bowl, whisk well the oil, juices and spices. Add salt and pepper to taste.
5. Add half of the green onions, half of parsley, currants, and nuts.
6. Toss with the cooled rice and let stand for at least 20 minutes.
7. If needed adjust seasoning with pepper and salt.
8. Garnish with remaining parsley and green onions.

Nutrition: Calories per serving: 450; Carbs: 50.0g; Protein: 9.0g; Fat: 24.0g

Orange, Dates And Asparagus On Quinoa Salad

Servings: 8 | Cooking: 25 min

Ingredients

- ¼ cup chopped pecans, toasted
- ½ cup white onion, finely chopped
- ½ jalapeno pepper, diced
- ½ lb. asparagus, sliced into 2-inch lengths, steamed and chilled
- ½ tsp salt
- 1 cup fresh orange sections
- 1 cup uncooked quinoa
- 1 tsp olive oil
- 2 cups water
- 2 tbsp minced red onion
- 5 dates, pitted and chopped
- ¼ tsp freshly ground black pepper
- ¼ tsp salt
- 1 garlic clove, minced
- 1 tbsp extra virgin olive oil
- 2 tbsp chopped fresh mint

- 2 tbsp fresh lemon juice
- Mint sprigs – optional

Directions

1. On medium high fire, place a large nonstick pan and heat 1 tsp oil.
2. Add white onion and sauté for two minutes.
3. Add quinoa and for 5 minutes sauté it.
4. Add salt and water. Bring to a boil, once boiling, slow fire to a simmer and cook for 15 minutes while covered.
5. Turn off fire and leave for 15 minutes, to let quinoa absorb the remaining water.
6. Transfer quinoa to a large salad bowl. Add jalapeno pepper, asparagus, dates, red onion, pecans and oranges. Toss to combine.
7. Make the dressing by mixing garlic, pepper, salt, olive oil and lemon juice in a small bowl.
8. Pour dressing into quinoa salad along with chopped mint, mix well.
9. If desired, garnish with mint sprigs before serving.

Nutrition: Calories: 265.2; Carbs: 28.3g; Protein: 14.6g; Fat: 10.4g

Stuffed Tomatoes With Green Chili

Servings: 6 | Cooking: 55 min

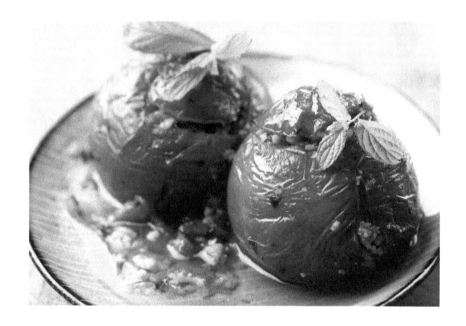

Ingredients

- 4 oz Colby-Jack shredded cheese
- ¼ cup water
- 1 cup uncooked quinoa
- 6 large ripe tomatoes
- ¼ tsp freshly ground black pepper
- ¾ tsp ground cumin
- 1 tsp salt, divided
- 1 tbsp fresh lime juice

- 1 tbsp olive oil
- 1 tbsp chopped fresh oregano
- 1 cup chopped onion
- 2 cups fresh corn kernels
- 2 poblano chilies

Directions

1. Preheat broiler to high.
2. Slice lengthwise the chilies and press on a baking sheet lined with foil. Broil for 8 minutes. Remove from oven and let cool for 10 minutes. Peel the chilies and chop coarsely and place in medium sized bowl.
3. Place onion and corn in baking sheet and broil for ten minutes. Stir two times while broiling. Remove from oven and mix in with chopped chilies.
4. Add black pepper, cumin, ¼ tsp salt, lime juice, oil and oregano. Mix well.
5. Cut off the tops of tomatoes and set aside. Leave the tomato shell intact as you scoop out the tomato pulp.
6. Drain tomato pulp as you press down with a spoon. Reserve 1 ¼ cups of tomato pulp liquid and

discard the rest. Invert the tomato shells on a wire rack for 30 mins and then wipe the insides dry with a paper towel.

7. Season with ½ tsp salt the tomato pulp.
8. On a sieve over a bowl, place quinoa. Add water until it covers quinoa. Rub quinoa grains for 30 seconds together with hands; rinse and drain. Repeat this procedure two times and drain well at the end.
9. In medium saucepan bring to a boil remaining salt, ¼ cup water, quinoa and tomato liquid.
10.   Once boiling, reduce heat and simmer for 15 minutes or until liquid is fully absorbed. Remove from heat and fluff quinoa with fork. Transfer and mix well the quinoa with the corn mixture.
11. Spoon ¾ cup of the quinoa-corn mixture into the tomato shells, top with cheese and cover with the tomato top. Bake in a preheated 350oF oven for 15 minutes and then broil high for another 1.5 minutes.

Nutrition: Calories per serving: 276; Carbs: 46.3g; Protein: 13.4g; Fat: 4.1g

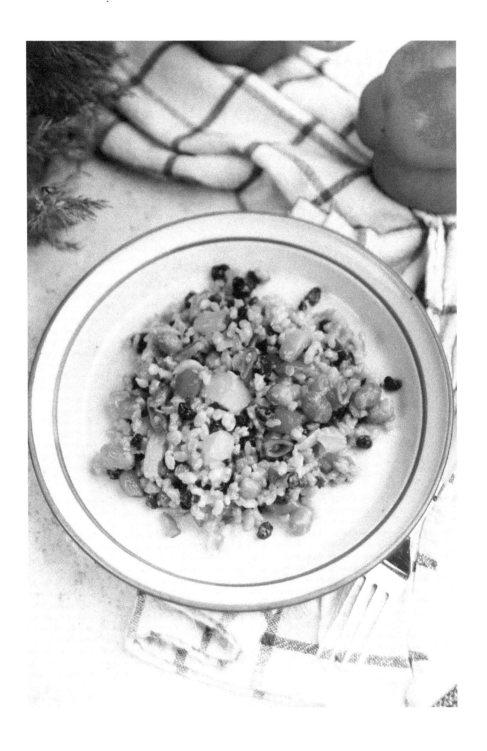

Chapter 7: Dessert Recipes

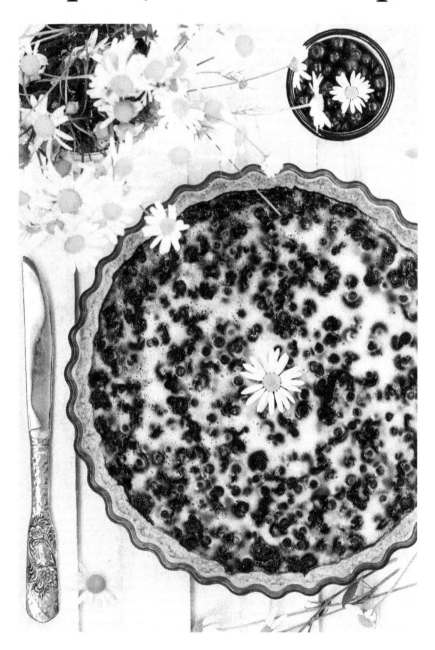

Creamy Pie

Servings: 6 | Cooking: 30 min

Ingredients

- ¼ cup lemon juice
- 1 cup cream
- 4 egg yolks
- 4 tablespoons Erythritol
- 1 tablespoon cornstarch
- 1 teaspoon vanilla extract
- 3 tablespoons butter
- 6 oz wheat flour, whole grain

Directions

1. Mix up together wheat flour and butter and knead the soft dough.
2. Put the dough in the round cake mold and flatten it in the shape of pie crust.
3. Bake it for 15 minutes at 365F.
4. Meanwhile, make the lemon filling: Mix up together cream, egg yolks, and lemon juice. When the liquid is smooth, start to heat it up over the medium heat. Stir it constantly.

5. When the liquid is hot, add vanilla extract, cornstarch, and Erythritol. Whisk well until smooth.
6. Brin the lemon filling to boil and remove it from the heat.
7. Cool it to the room temperature.
8. Cook the pie crust to the room temperature.
9. Pour the lemon filling over the pie crust, flatten it well and leave to cool in the fridge for 25 minutes.

Nutrition: calories 225; fat 11.4; fiber 0.8; carbs 34.8; protein 5.2

Hazelnut Pudding

Servings: 8 | Cooking: 40 min

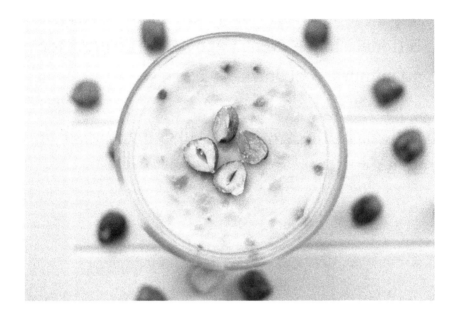

Ingredients

- 2 and ¼ cups almond flour
- 3 tablespoons hazelnuts, chopped
- 5 eggs, whisked
- 1 cup stevia
- 1 and 1/3 cups Greek yogurt
- 1 teaspoon baking powder
- 1 teaspoon vanilla extract

Directions

1. In a bowl, combine the flour with the hazelnuts and the other ingredients, whisk well, and pour into a cake pan lined with parchment paper,
2. Introduce in the oven at 350 degrees F, bake for 30 minutes, cool down, slice and serve.

Nutrition: calories 178; fat 8.4; fiber 8.2; carbs 11.5; protein 1.4

Mediterranean Cheesecakes

Servings: 1 Cheesecake | Cooking: 20 min

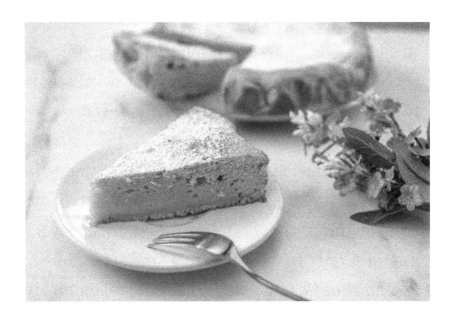

Ingredients

- 4 cups shredded phyllo (kataifi dough)
- 1/2 cup butter, melted
- 12 oz. cream cheese
- 1 cup Greek yogurt
- 3/4 cup confectioners' sugar
- 1 TB. vanilla extract
- 2 TB. orange blossom water
- 1 TB. orange zest

- 2 large eggs
- 1 cup coconut flakes

Directions

1. Preheat the oven to 450°F.
2. In a large bowl, and using your hands, combine shredded phyllo and melted butter, working the two together and breaking up phyllo shreds as you work.
3. Using a 12-cup muffin tin, add 1/3 cup shredded phyllo mixture to each tin, and press down to form crust on the bottom of the cup. Bake crusts for 8 minutes, remove from the oven, and set aside.
4. In a large bowl, and using an electric mixer on low speed, blend cream cheese and Greek yogurt for 1 minute.
5. Add confectioners' sugar, vanilla extract, orange blossom water, and orange zest, and blend 1 minute.
6. Add eggs, and blend for about 30 seconds or just until eggs are incorporated.
7. Lightly coat the sides of each muffin tin with cooking spray.
8. Pour about 1/3 cup cream cheese mixture over crust in each tin. Do not overflow.

9. Bake for 12 minutes.

10. Spread shredded coconut on a baking sheet, and place in the oven with cheesecakes to toast for 4 or 5 minutes or until golden brown. Remove from the oven, and set aside.

11. Remove cheesecakes from the oven, and cool for 1 hour on the countertop.

12. Place the tin in the refrigerator, and cool for 1 more hour.

13. To serve, dip a sharp knife in warm water and then run it along the sides of cheesecakes to loosen from the tin. Gently remove cheesecakes and place on a serving plate.

14. Sprinkle with toasted coconut flakes, and serve.

Melon Cucumber Smoothie

Servings: 2 | Cooking: 5 min

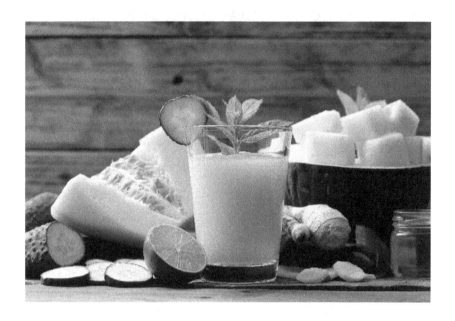

Ingredients

- ½ cucumber
- 2 slices of melon
- 2 tablespoons lemon juice
- 1 pear, peeled and sliced
- 3 fresh mint leaves
- ½ cup almond milk

Directions

1. Place all Ingredients: in a blender.

2. Blend until smooth.

3. Pour in a glass container and allow to chill in the fridge for at least 30 minutes.

Nutrition: Calories per serving: 253; Carbs: 59.3g; Protein: 5.7g; Fat: 2.1g

Mediterranean Style Fruit Medley

Servings: 7 | Cooking: 5 min

Ingredients

- 4 fuyu persimmons, sliced into wedges
- 1 ½ cups grapes, halved
- 8 mint leaves, chopped
- 1 tablespoon lemon juice
- 1 tablespoon honey
- ½ cups almond, toasted and chopped

Directions

1. Combine all Ingredients: in a bowl.
2. Toss then chill before serving.

Nutrition: Calories per serving:159; Carbs: 32g; Protein: 3g; Fat: 4g

CPSIA information can be obtained
at www.ICGtesting.com
Printed in the USA
BVIIW092310210621
610124BV00010B/2061

9 781911 688983